Pocket Guide to Practical Psychopharmacology

Andrea Fagiolini
Alessandro Cuomo
Roger S. McIntyre

Pocket Guide to Practical Psychopharmacology

Lithium and Anticonvulsants in Psychiatric Practice

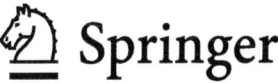 Springer

Andrea Fagiolini
Department of Molecular Medicine
University of Siena
Siena, Siena, Italy

Alessandro Cuomo
Department of Molecular Medicine
University of Siena
Siena, Siena, Italy

Roger S. McIntyre
University Health Network, MP
9-325
University of Toronto
Toronto, ON, Canada

ISBN 978-3-030-98059-7   ISBN 978-3-030-98060-3   (eBook)
https://doi.org/10.1007/978-3-030-98060-3

This Springer imprint is published by the registered company Springer Nature
Switzerland AG
The registered company address is: Gewerbestrasse 11, 6330 Cham, Switzerland

Preface

This booklet is intended to provide an accessible and practical reference for psychiatric residents and for any other healthcare practitioner seeking for a tool that is simple, concise, and immediately useful for everyday clinical practice. The information is ready to use, easy to remember, and focused primarily on clinically relevant issues, such as preliminary laboratory evaluations, drug dosages, schedules, indications, contraindications, side effects, and strategies to manage them.

The use of classic mood stabilizers (e.g., lithium, valproate, and carbamazepine) is discussed and examined in its practicalities through the presentation of a clinical case for each of the three medications, with the goal of reflecting clinical practice in the "real world" management with mood stabilizers of patients with bipolar disorder.

Siena, Italy   Andrea Fagiolini
Siena, Italy   Alessandro Cuomo
Toronto, ON, Canada   Roger S. McIntyre

Contents

Lithium

1.1 Clinical Case: Marco, a Patient with Bipolar Depression

Marco is a 26-year-old Caucasian male, graduate student, presents to the outpatient unit complaining profound sadness, tiredness, inability to enjoy the things he used to enjoy, difficulty concentrating, ideas that life is not worth living, mild agitation, distractibility, and indecisiveness. He has lost all interest in sex and going out socializing. He watches TV until very late finding it difficult to fall asleep thereafter. In the morning, he feels tired, exhausted and tends to lie in bed till the afternoon.

1.2 Family History

Father: No personal or family history of major psychiatric diseases, except for a likely depression and social anxiety disorder experienced by his grandmother.

Mother: Suffers from bipolar disorder type 2, presently and successfully treated with lithium.

Sister 1: Suffers from panic disorder and major depressive disorder but is currently well, on paroxetine 20 mg/day.

Sister 2: No history of any psychiatric disorders.

A. Fagiolini et al., *Pocket Guide to Practical Psychopharmacology*, https://doi.org/10.1007/978-3-030-98060-3_1

1.3   Clinical History

Marco reports one previous episode of depression, about 6 years earlier, with symptoms that were similar to those that he is presently experiencing. He states that the episode was not treated, as it resolved spontaneously, when he was "forced" to go on a family vacation to the Caribbean.

He states that his symptoms cleared very quickly. He went to sleep depressed and woke up full of energy, enthusiastic, extroverted, sociable, full of confidence, enthusiasm, and energy. He also reported trouble controlling his temper and to have spent a few days shouting at people and starting arguments or fights even over minor matters. He was arrested because of driving recklessly and speeding and then brought to the hospital, treated with medications he does not remember of, and then discharged. He took no medication since, until this current episode, which started about 3 weeks ago.

1.4   Physical and Mental State Examination

Weight: 80 kg
   Height: 182 cm
   Physical examination is unremarkable apart from tachycardia of 95/min. He is casually dressed, establishes a good rapport and is cooperative. He appears somewhat fidgety and restless but not severely agitated. Periodically, he gets tearful, and his voice becomes tremulous. He does not have any formal thought disorder psychotic symptoms. He has good insight into her symptoms. He reports fleeting thoughts that life is not worth living and admits to having thought about suicide a couple of times in the past years but denies any current suicide plan or intent and contracts for safety. He acknowledges that he should have sought help earlier but expresses his willingness to start treatment now.

1.5   We Decide to Consider Starting Treatment with Lithium

1.5.1   What are the Indications of Lithium?

In most countries, lithium is indicated for:

- Treatment of manic episodes of bipolar disorder
- Maintenance treatment of bipolar disorder

1.5.2   What are the Contraindications of Lithium?

- Hypersensitivity to inactive ingredients used in the lithium carbonate formulations (tablet, capsule) or lithium citrate formulations
- Severe renal disease, cardiovascular conditions, dehydration, or sodium insufficiency

1.5.3   What are the Warnings of Lithium?

Lithium toxicity is closely related to serum lithium levels and can occur at doses that are close to therapeutic levels. Facilities for prompt and accurate serum lithium determinations should be available before initiating therapy.

1.6   Clinical Considerations

Marco is presently experiencing a depressive episode. However, he has a history of at least one manic episode and hence fulfils a diagnosis of bipolar I disorder.

We decided to consider lithium as he has no apparent contraindications, because of lithium's mood stabilizing efficacy and because of lithium's ability to decrease suicide risk. We decided to not immediately start an antidepressant. In our experience, a subpopulation of patients with bipolar disorder may need an antidepressant. However, the antidepressant should not be started until the patient is adequately treated with a mood stabilizer and/or an atypical antipsychotic and until the possibility that depression responds to monotherapy with a mood stabilizer alone and/or an atypical antipsychotic (i.e., responds to an anti-manic agent, without an antidepressant) has been ruled out.

1.7   What is the Mechanism of Action of Lithium?

The exact mechanism of action of lithium is unknown. However, lithium is believed to have the capacity to reduce dopamine receptor hypersensitivity and to stimulate serotonin and norepinephrine activity. Lithium is also known to decrease glycogen synthase kinase 3 (GSK-3) concentrations which indirectly modulates neurotransmission across many different neurochemicals. By reducing inositol monophosphatase, lithium is involved in intracellular second-messenger pathways.

Other possible mechanisms of lithium include:

- Normalization of low cerebrospinal fluid
- Normalization of low γ-aminobutyric acid (GABA)
- Neurotrophic effects by enhanced neurogenesis
- Antioxidant properties and prevention of neural apoptosis
- Neuroprotective effects by stimulating production of brain-derived neurotrophic factor (BDNF) in patients with chronic lithium treatment

1.8   Which Laboratory Tests would you Order for Marco?

Before initiation of treatment with lithium, it is recommended to obtain patient's thorough medical history and perform baseline evaluations and laboratory test, such as:

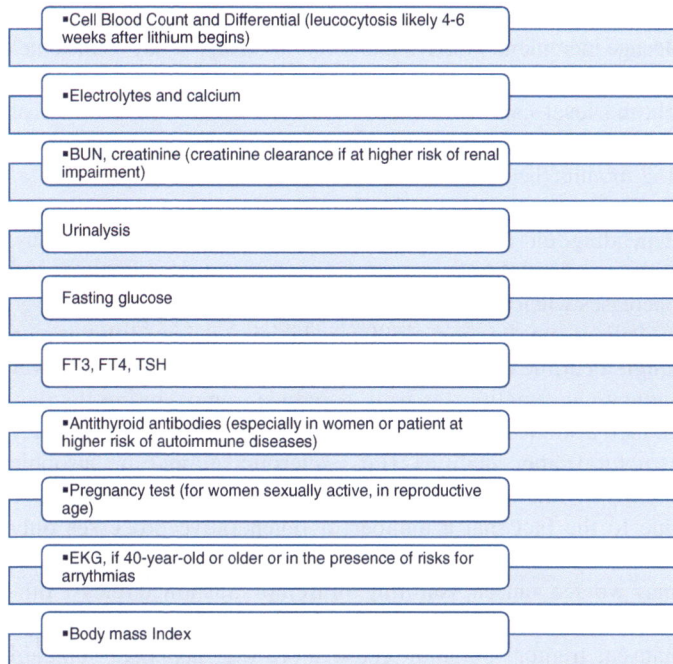

- Cell Blood Count and Differential (leucocytosis likely 4-6 weeks after lithium begins)

- Electrolytes and calcium

- BUN, creatinine (creatinine clearance if at higher risk of renal impairment)

Urinalysis

Fasting glucose

FT3, FT4, TSH

- Antithyroid antibodies (especially in women or patient at higher risk of autoimmune diseases)

- Pregnancy test (for women sexually active, in reproductive age)

- EKG, if 40-year-old or older or in the presence of risks for arrythmias

- Body mass Index

Marco's laboratory tests are all within normal limits.

1.8.1   Which Dose Would You Prescribe?

We decided to start Marco on 300 mg twice a day (b.i.d). For healthy patients with more severe symptoms, we sometime begin lithium at three times a day (t.i.d.).

1.9   How Would You Monitor Marco's Tolerability?

Patients must be closely monitored for side effects. A 12-h lithium plasma level must be obtained 2–5 days (depending on the starting dose and on the patient's kidney function) after starting lithium. Thereafter, the dose can be increased every 2–4 days.

Lithium blood level should be checked 3–5 days after each dosage increment. Steady-state levels arise in 4–5 days, but sometimes take up to 7 days. Once a stable dose is achieved, lithium plasma level can be obtained weekly-biweekly (first month of treatment), every 2–3 weeks (second month of treatment) or every 1–2 months (beginning the fourth month of treatment).

The targeted lithium blood level should be 0.5–1.2 mEq/L depending on age, tolerability, response, and clinical status. Lithium tolerability is greater during the acute manic phase and decreases when manic symptoms subside.

Patients on dosages <1500 mg/day may receive lithium on a single bedtime dose. This may produce less polyuria and fewer kidney abnormalities as well as reduce tremor during the day. In fact, a single (qd), bedtime dosing often results in less kidney structural abnormalities (i.e., sclerotic glomeruli, atrophic tubuli, or interstitial fibrosis) and less polyuria. This may be due to the fact that a number of regenerative processes only occur in periods with low lithium concentrations. However, this may worsen nausea, vomiting, or tremor. Sustained release lithium may lower side effects related to peak concentrations (e.g., nausea, tremor) but may cause more diarrhea than standard lithium. Lithium citrate may have fewer GI and allergic side effects.

Marco did not show any severe side effect.

1.10   When Would You Repeat the Laboratory Tests?

Plasma level is usually measured 2–5 days after introducing lithium, then once a week in first 2–3 weeks, and later once in 1–2 months.

Plasma levels should be assessed in case of dosage increase, co-medication, or presence of adverse effects (i.e., vomit or diarrhea) or toxicity.

The blood sample for plasma level monitoring should be taken 12 h (security interval 10–14 h) after the previous drug dose. In patients receiving once-daily administration, the serum concentration at 24 h should serve as the control value.

As steady-state concentrations are reached in approximately 4 days after lithium initiation, mood stabilizing effects may be expected within 5–7 days, and may take longer before they reach their maximum effect.

When rapid treatment of acute mania is required, antipsychotic agent may be preferred as an alternative to lithium or combined with lithium.

- Electrolytes and calcium should be reassessed at least after 1–2 weeks, then every 3–4 weeks for the first 2 months and then every 3–6 months depending on clinical status. Laboratory tests should be repeated more frequently if patients experience symptoms such as dizziness, clumsiness, ataxia, apathy, dysphoria, blurred vision, diarrhoea, loss of appetite, nausea, vomiting, constipation, abdominal pain, excessive need to drink fluids, increased urination, tiredness, weakness, muscle pain, confusion, disorientation, difficulty thinking, headaches, etc. Check lithium levels immediately if any severe physical symptom occur or whenever the patient has severe nausea or vomiting.
- Renal function should be reassessed after 1 month and then every 2–3 months in first 6 months of lithium treatment; after that, tests should be repeated every 3–6 months.
- Thyroid function should be assessed once or twice in first 6 months of lithium treatment; after that, tests should be repeated in 6–12 months.

Marco's laboratory tests continued to be within normal limits and he achieved a blood concentration of 0.78 mmol/L with a dose of 1200 mg/day. His symptoms started to improve after about 1 week and continued improving thereafter.

1.11   How Would You Manage Marco's Lithium During Maintenance Treatment?

Usually, doses range between 600 mg and 1800 mg (0.6–1.0 mmol/L). Most often, the maintenance dose is around 900–1200 mg/day. Lithium dosage must be individualized according to serum levels and clinical response. After stabilization, some patients prefer taking lithium in a single daily dose, usually at night. Marco should receive education about the possibility of a change in lithium level after dietary changes, particularly those involving caffeine and salt, with a consequent increase in the risk of developing lithium toxicity. A decrease in sodium or caffeine intake may result in higher serum lithium levels.

When possible decreasing lithium dosage as close as clinically possible to 0.6 mmol/l during prophylaxis often reduces morbidity and side effects. In the case of Marco, we decided to wait at least 4–5 months before attempting to reduce the dose.

1.12   What if Marco Was an Older Patient?

For elderly patients, lithium treatment should start with 150–300 mg/day, and continue with 300–1200 mg/day, depending on tolerability and blood levels.

1.13   What are the Strategies to Safely Use Lithium in Late Life Patients?

- Careful plasma levels monitoring of lithium is necessary for elderly patients
- Comorbidity and drug interactions should be carefully considered, given the possible interactions between lithium and drugs prescribed to the elderly (e.g., diuretics).
- Special consideration should be taken in patients with renal failure, who might be at greater risk of toxicity due to impaired drug elimination. Lithium increases the risk of renal dysfunction if administered in elderly
- Elderly patients are usually treated with lowest recommended drug doses
- Neuroprotective features of lithium may have positive effects and prevent cognitive decline in elderly.

1.14   Can Lithium Be Used in Children and Adolescents?

Besides therapeutic effects, lithium also reduces risk of suicide, and it has been used in children and adolescents with bipolar disorder. The evidence for treatment of pediatric bipolar disorder with lithium is relatively small, but recent data has enabled lithium to re-emerge as a valuable treatment. Using lithium in children is challenging, given the narrow therapeutic window and the many potential side effects. However, the efficacy of lithium for many symptoms of bipolar disorder, including suicidality, continues to suggest an important place for this medication in the treatment armamentarium of child psychiatry.

Common or worrisome adverse effects of treatment with lithium in pediatric population may include gastrointestinal, endocrine or renal dysfunction, as well as many of the other side effects that have been described for adult patients.

1.15   Can Lithium Be Used in Pregnant Patients?

Lithium use is associated with increased risk of cardiovascular abnormalities, particularly in the offspring of women who were taking the medication during the first trimester of pregnancy. Recent data suggest that this risk is lower than previously considered but still worth of being considered when the risk/benefit ratio of lithium treatment has to be evaluated in a woman who is about to start a pregnancy.

Lithium administration during pregnancy may increase risk of neonatal complications.

Breastfeeding while undergoing lithium treatment is not recommended because of risk of toxicity of an infant.

1.16   What Would the Dose Be if Marco Had a Renal Disease?

Usually, alternative medications are recommended for patients with kidney disease. However, there may be patients whose risk/benefit ratio for lithium remains favorable even in the presence of renal disease, e.g., patients at very high risk of suicide. For patients with renal disease, it is usually necessary to prescribe:

- 50–70% of standard dose if creatinine clearance is 10–50 mL/min.
- 25–50% of standard dose if creatinine clearance is below 10 mL/min.

A frequent evaluation of lithium blood levels is necessary.

1.17   What is the Pharmacokinetic Profile of Lithium?

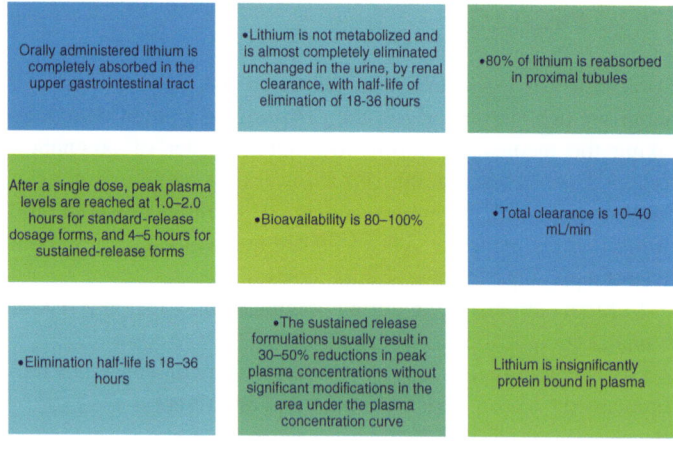

Orally administered lithium is completely absorbed in the upper gastrointestinal tract

- Lithium is not metabolized and is almost completely eliminated unchanged in the urine, by renal clearance, with half-life of elimination of 18-36 hours

- 80% of lithium is reabsorbed in proximal tubules

After a single dose, peak plasma levels are reached at 1.0–2.0 hours for standard-release dosage forms, and 4–5 hours for sustained-release forms

- Bioavailability is 80–100%

- Total clearance is 10–40 mL/min

- Elimination half-life is 18–36 hours

- The sustained release formulations usually result in 30–50% reductions in peak plasma concentrations without significant modifications in the area under the plasma concentration curve

Lithium is insignificantly protein bound in plasma

Marco is physically healthy and is not taking other medications. What if he was taking other medications?

Lithium levels are increased by medications such as	• **Angiotensin-converting enzyme inhibitors such as enalapril and captopril, and angiotensin II receptor antagonists, such as losartan** • **Diuretics (e.g., thiazide), except potassium and sodium sparing diuretics** • **NSAIDS (30–61% increase),** • **Other substances and medications such as alcohol, albuterol, ampicillin, discontinuation of caffeine, ketamine, marijuana, mazindol, methyldopa, metronidazole, phenytoin, spectinomycin, and succinylcholine.**
Lithium levels are decreased by medications such as	• Acetazolamide • Bronchodilators • Caffeine • Corticosteroids • Carbonic anhydrase inhibitors • Xanthine diuretics • Sodium bicarbonate • Theophylline • DHEA

Patients at steady state on thiazide diuretic or salt restricted diet can have lithium added safely if the doses of both medications are not changed without appropriate monitoring of blood levels. Potassium and sodium sparing diuretics have minimal or no effect on lithium levels.

The concurrent use of calcium channel blocking agents with lithium may increase the risk of neurotoxicity, with symptoms like ataxia, diarrhea, nausea, tinnitus, tremors, and/or vomiting.

Despite being frequently combined with anticonvulsant agents, the risk of adverse effects may be increased. Combination of lithium and **valproate** has greater possibility of various side effects including weight gain, tremor, or sedation. Lithium combined with **carbamazepine** has greater risk of neurotoxicity. Lithium in combination with second-generation **antipsychotics** may contribute to neurological alteration.

However, in our experience, the balance between risks and benefits of the above combinations with valproate, carbamazepine, or antipsychotics is often favorable for patients who do not respond to monotherapy.

The above is just a general summary. If a medication is not reported above, this does not mean that there is no interaction. In those cases, please consult the PDR/appropriate literature carefully.

1.18 What are the Adverse Effects that You Would Monitor in a Patient Like Marco?

Adverse reactions are usually related to high serum lithium concentrations or to individual patient sensitivity to lithium.

Common initial side effects may include hand tremor (present at rest, but usually get worse on intentional movement), dyspepsia, diarrhea, polyuria, polydipsia, urinary frequency, nausea, and dizziness. Common later side effects include thirst, polyuria, weight gain, edema, acne, leukocytosis, cloudy thinking, and hair loss (more frequent in women).

Many adverse effects require lithium discontinuation but many other can be managed by reducing the dose, escalating the dose more slowly, changing the time of administration, or changing the lithium preparation (e.g., switching from normal release to slow release or vice versa).

For instance:

- **Mild tremor** may be diminished by:
  - Switching to time-sustained preparation
  - Changing time of administration to single q.h.s. dose
  - Changing time of administration to a more frequent, smaller dose
  - Decreasing daily dose/lithium level

- Propranolol → DO NOT PRESCRIBE if: bronchospasm, asthma, congestive heart failure, or other contraindications to beta blockers. Dose of propranolol depends on age of the patient.
- **Nausea** may be diminished by:
  - Diminishing lithium dose/level
  - Spreading out lithium dose
  - Ingestion of lithium with food or milk
  - Switching to sustained release preparation (Note: this may increase the risk of diarrhea)
- **Diarrhea** can be diminished by:
  - Switching from slow release to normal release lithium
  - Switching from b.i.d. to single q.h.s. dose
  - Making diet adjustments (e.g., avoiding caffeine or food that may increase the risk of diarrhea)
- **Polyuria/polydipsia/nephrogenic diabetes insipidus** (urine > 3 liters/day) is usually due to reduced response to vasopressin antidiuretic hormone (ADH), with difficulty concentrating urine and maintaining serum lithium level, and often results in increased sodium and decreased potassium levels. It can be diminished by:
  - Switching to lithium once a day, single q.h.s. dose. Usually, q.h.s. doses are better tolerated but this may cause nocturnal enuresis.
  - Lowering dose/level.
  - Adding potassium 20–40 mEq/L, if there are not medical contraindications.
  - Prescribing K-Na sparing diuretics like amiloride 5–10 mg/day or spironolactone, if no medical contraindication.
  - Avoiding hydrochlorothiazides: May increase plasma sodium, further decrease serum potassium and increase plasma lithium levels by 30–50%. If thiazides are necessary, may combine thiazide with amiloride to prevent hypokalemia.

- Prescribing ibuprofen or indometacin, if no medical contra-indications. Given that NSAIDs increase plasma lithium 30–60% in 3–10 days, a very close monitoring of lithium level and appropriate adjustments in lithium dose are required if these medications are prescribed.
- **Tubulo-interstitial nephritis/kidney insufficiency** often requires considering lithium discontinuation:
  - If creatinine level is greater than 1.6 mg/100 ml, consult a nephrologist and consider discontinuing lithium while problem is potentially reversible. Discontinuation has to be weighted against increased risk of suicide, especially in the first year after lithium discontinuation.
- **Hypothyroidism**
  - It is often possible to continue lithium. May consider adding thyroxine.
- **Hyperparathyroidism**
  - Symptoms of hyperparathyroidism include ataxia, apathy, dysphoria, loss of appetite, nausea, vomiting, constipation, abdominal, pain, need to drink more fluids, increased urination, tiredness, weakness, muscle pain, confusion, disorientation, difficulty thinking, headaches, depression and mood changes, apathy, convulsions.
  - Check PTH and calcium levels (hypercalcemia).
- **Acne:**
  - May try antibiotics and/or retinoic acid. May be necessary to reduce or stop lithium.
- **Psoriasis:**
  - Lithium may worsen pre-existing or subclinical psoriasis.
  - Consider lowering lithium dose, refer to a dermatologist.
  - Discontinue lithium if psoriasis is severe or systemic.
- **Weight gain**
  - Relatively common.
  - Edema may also contribute.

- May be related to hypothyroidism, insulin-like effects on carbohydrate metabolism, increased intake of high calorie beverages.
- Early referral to nutritionist is advised.
- **Cardiovascular** side effects may result in EKG changes, which frequently include:
  - T-wave flattening, T-wave inversion, widening of QRS complex. Usually, these EKG changes are benign, reversable, and should not be confused with more serious issues such as hypokalemia (check potassium level).
  - At toxic level, lithium may produce S-T segment depression and Q-T interval prolongation.
  - Arrhythmias more often occur in patients with pre-existing cardiac diseases (check EKG prior to starting lithium if a heart disease is suspected).
  - Sino-atrial node dysfunction is common and may cause dizziness, fainting, and palpitations.
  - Ventricular arrhythmias are rare but sudden deaths have been reported, most often in patients with pre-existing heart disease.
  - Consult a cardiologist before placing on lithium a patient with pre-existing cardiovascular problems.

1.19   What if Marco Develops Fever or Vomit?

In case of fever or vomiting: temporarily stop lithium, immediately check blood levels.

1.20   What if Marco Develops Toxicity? What Are the First Signs?

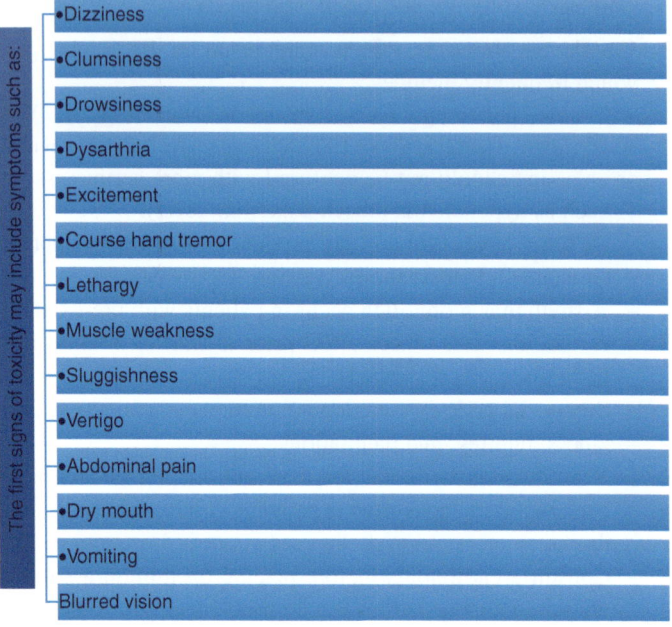

The first signs of toxicity may include symptoms such as:
- Dizziness
- Clumsiness
- Drowsiness
- Dysarthria
- Excitement
- Course hand tremor
- Lethargy
- Muscle weakness
- Sluggishness
- Vertigo
- Abdominal pain
- Dry mouth
- Vomiting
- Blurred vision

The toxic concentrations for lithium (≥ 1.5 mEq/L) are close to the therapeutic range (0.6–1.2 mEq/L). Lithium may take up to 24 h to distribute into the tissues, so occurrence of acute toxicity symptoms may be delayed. Severe reactions are most often seen at levels of 2.0 mEq/L and above.

1.21   Which Factors May Increase the Risks of Lithium Toxicity?

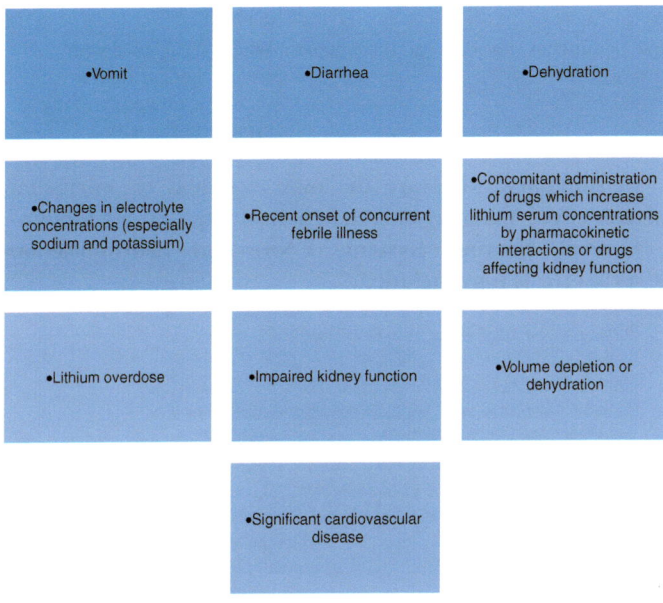

1.22   Which Other Recommendations Should Be Provided to Patients Taking Lithium?

Patients should be frequently reminded that lithium retention might occur in case of dehydration or excessive sodium loss.

Patient recommendation	
Consume stable amounts of fluids and salt	Avoid excessive exercise
Avoid working heavily in hot weather	Avoid starting diets before discussing them with your doctor
Discontinue lithium and contact a pharmacotherapist in case of symptoms of possible toxicity (e.g., vomiting or fever or other signs of toxicity)	Contact a pharmacotherapist in case you start new medications

Patient recommendation	
Tell any doctor that you consult with, about taking lithium	Lithium level should always be assessed in case of diarrhea
Use of diuretics should be careful to avoid toxicity	When is combined with antipsychotics, lithium should be titrated carefully to avoid neurotoxicity

In summary, what are the most common or worrisome adverse effects that may be seen in patients treated with lithium?

Central Nervous System (CNS) and neuromuscular adverse effects may include:

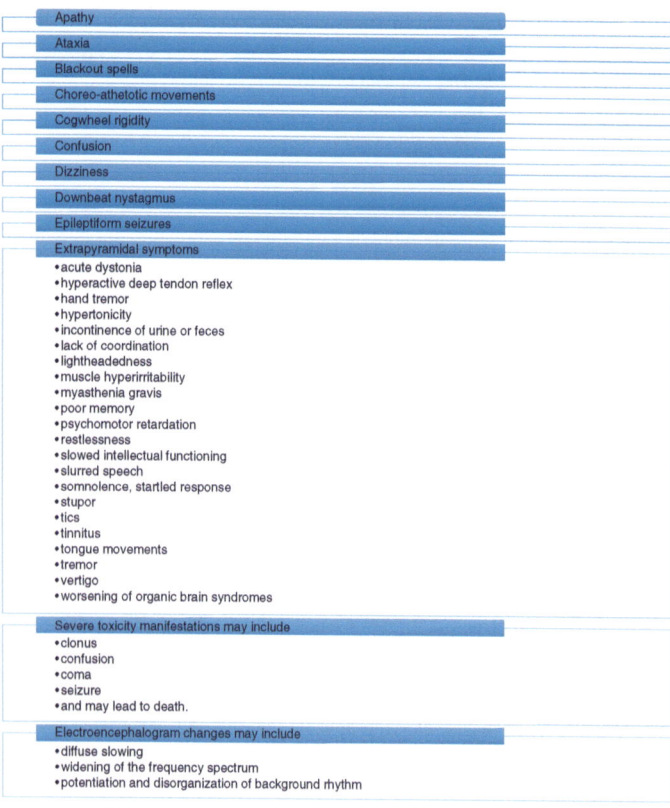

Apathy

Ataxia

Blackout spells

Choreo-athetotic movements

Cogwheel rigidity

Confusion

Dizziness

Downbeat nystagmus

Epileptiform seizures

Extrapyramidal symptoms
- acute dystonia
- hyperactive deep tendon reflex
- hand tremor
- hypertonicity
- incontinence of urine or feces
- lack of coordination
- lightheadedness
- muscle hyperirritability
- myasthenia gravis
- poor memory
- psychomotor retardation
- restlessness
- slowed intellectual functioning
- slurred speech
- somnolence, startled response
- stupor
- tics
- tinnitus
- tongue movements
- tremor
- vertigo
- worsening of organic brain syndromes

Severe toxicity manifestations may include
- clonus
- confusion
- coma
- seizure
- and may lead to death.

Electroencephalogram changes may include
- diffuse slowing
- widening of the frequency spectrum
- potentiation and disorganization of background rhythm

Cases of pseudotumor cerebri (increased intracranial pressure and papilledema) have been reported with lithium use. Pseudotumor cerebri may result in constriction of visual fields, enlargement of the blind spot, and eventual blindness due to optic atrophy. Lithium should be discontinued, if clinically possible, if this syndrome occurs.

An encephalopathic syndrome (characterized by lethargy, fever, tremulousness and confusion, extrapyramidal symptoms, weakness, leukocytosis, elevated serum enzymes, BUN and FBS) has occurred in a limited number of patients treated with lithium plus an antipsychotic. In some of these cases, the syndrome was followed by irreversible brain damage. Patients receiving such combined therapy should be monitored closely for neurologic toxicity and treatment discontinued promptly if such signs appear.

Cardiovascular adverse effects may include:

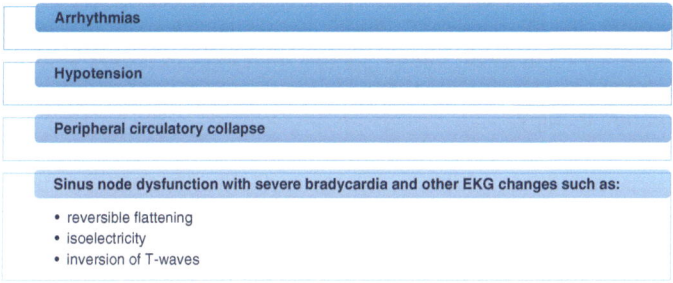

- Arrhythmias
- Hypotension
- Peripheral circulatory collapse
- Sinus node dysfunction with severe bradycardia and other EKG changes such as:
  - reversible flattening
  - isoelectricity
  - inversion of T-waves

A possible association between treatment with lithium and the unmasking of Brugada syndrome has been reported. Lithium should generally be avoided in patients suspected of having Brugada syndrome. Consultation with a cardiologist is recommended before starting lithium if a patient has risk factors for Brugada syndrome, e.g., unexplained syncope or palpitations, or a family history of Brugada syndrome, or a family history of sudden unexplained death before the age of 45 years.

Gastrointestinal adverse effects may include: anorexia, nausea, vomiting, diarrhea, gastritis, salivary gland swelling, abdominal pain, excessive salivation, flatulence, vomiting.

Genitourinary adverse effects may include: glycosuria, decreased creatinine clearance, albuminuria, oliguria, and renal failure.

Chronic lithium treatment may be associated with diminution of kidney concentrating ability, occasionally presenting as nephrogenic diabetes insipidus, with polyuria (urine concentrating defect), polydipsia, and thirst. In these cases, patients should be carefully treated to avoid dehydration, lithium retention, and toxicity. This condition is often reversible when lithium is discontinued.

Nephrotic syndrome with minimal change disease and focal segmental glomerulosclerosis, has also been reported. Discontinuation of lithium usually results in remission of nephrotic syndrome.

Morphologic changes with glomerular and interstitial fibrosis and nephron atrophy may be observed after long-term chronic lithium therapy. However, morphologic changes have also been seen in patients with bipolar disease that have never exposed to lithium. Kidney function should be assessed before and during lithium therapy.

Dermatologic adverse effects: Drying and thinning of hair, alopecia, anesthesia of skin, acne, chronic folliculitis, xerosis cutis, psoriasis or its exacerbation, generalized pruritus with or without rash, cutaneous ulcers, angioedema.

Autonomic: Blurred vision, dry mouth, impotence/sexual dysfunction.

Thyroid Abnormalities: Euthyroid goiter and/or hypothyroidism (including myxedema) accompanied by lower T_3 and T_4. I^{131} uptake may be elevated. Paradoxically, rare cases of hyperthyroidism have been reported. Hyperparathyroidism and hypothyroidism may persist after lithium discontinuation.

Miscellaneous adverse effects: transient scotomata, exophthalmos, dehydration, weight loss, leukocytosis, headache, transient hyperglycemia, hypercalcemia, hyperparathyroidism, excessive weight gain, edematous swelling of ankles or wrists, metallic taste, dysgeusia/taste distortion, salty taste, thirst, swollen lips, tightness in chest, swollen and/or painful joints, fever, polyarthralgia, dental caries.

The development of painful discoloration of fingers and toes and coldness of the extremities within one day of the starting of treatment with lithium has been reported. The mechanism through which these symptoms (resembling Raynaud's syndrome) developed is not known.

Diarrhea, drowsiness, muscular weakness, vomiting, and lack of coordination may be early signs of lithium intoxication, and can occur at lithium levels below 2.0 mEq/L.

At higher blood levels, ataxia, giddiness, tinnitus, blurred vision, and a large output of dilute urine may be seen. Serum lithium levels above 3.0 mEq/L may produce a complex clinical picture, involving multiple organs and organ systems.

1.23 What Happens if Marco Abruptly Discontinues Lithium?

Abrupt discontinuation of lithium, even in symptom-free patients may lead to mania or depression relapse.

Rapid discontinuation may also cause other symptoms such as anxiety and emotional instability and **may increase suicide risk.**

Further Reading

Baird-Gunning J, Lea-Henry T, Hoegberg L, Gosselin S, Roberts DM. Lithium poisoning. J Intensive Care Med. 2016:1–15.

Coppen A, Abou-Saleh M, Milln P, Bailey J, Wood K. Decreasing lithium dosage reduces morbidity and side-effects during prophylaxis. J Affect Disord. 1983;5:353–62.

De Fazio P, Gaetano R, Caroleo M, et al. Lithium in late-life mania: a systematic review. Neuropsychiatr Dis Treat. 2017;2017(13):755–66.

Eskalith, Lithium carbonate FDA prescribing information. Last accessed on Sept 10, 2022, https://www.accessdata.fda.gov/drugsatfda_docs/label/20 04/16860slr074,18152slr020_eskalith_lbl.pdf

Gitlin M. Lithium side effects and toxicity: prevalence and management strategies. Int J Bipolar Disord. 2016;4(1):27.

Grandjean EM, Aubry JM. Lithium: updated human knowledge using an evidence-based approach. Part II: clinical pharmacology and therapeutic monitoring. CNS Drugs. 2009;23(4):331–49.

Grant B, Salpekar JA. Using lithium in children and adolescents with bipolar disorder: efficacy, tolerability, and practical considerations. Paediatr Drugs. 2018;20(4):303–14.

Hedya SA, Avula A, Swoboda HD. Lithium toxicity. In: StatPearls [Internet]. Treasure Island (FL): StatPearls Publishing; 2019. https://www.ncbi.nlm.nih.gov/books/NBK499992/.

Kamali M, Krishnamurthy VB, Baweja R, Saunders E, Gelenberg AJ. Lithium. In: Schatzberg A, Nemeroff C, editors. The American Psychiatric Association Publishing Textbook of Psychopharmacology. 5th ed. Washington (DC): The American Psychiatric Association Publishing; 2017. https://doi.org/10.1176/appi.books.9781615371624.

Lithium, FDA prescribing information. Last accessed on Sept 10, 2022, https://www.accessdata.fda.gov/drugsatfda_docs/label/2018/017812s033,018421s032,018558s027lbl.pdf and https://www.accessdata.fda.gov/drugsatfda_docs/label/2011/017812s028,018421s027lbl.pdf

Lithobid, Lithium carbonate extended release tablets, FDA prescribing information. Last accessed on Sept 10, 2022, https://www.accessdata.fda.gov/drugsatfda_docs/label/2020/018027s067lbl.pdf

Malhi GS, Tanious M, Das P, Coulston CM, Berk M. Potential mechanisms of action of lithium in bipolar disorder. Current understanding. CNS Drugs. 2013;27(2):135–53. https://doi.org/10.1007/s40263-013-0039-0.

Jerrold S. Maxmen, Sydney H. Kennedy, and Roger S. McIntyre. Psychotropic drugs fast facts (4th edition). WW Norton & Co., New York, New York, 2008, 260 pages, ISBN: 978-0393-20529.

Plengee P, Mellerwt T, Bolwigc G, Brun O, Hetmar JL, Larsena N, Rafaelsen OJ. Lithium treatment: does the kidney prefer one daily dose instead of two? Acta Psychiatr Scand. 1982;66:121–8.

Poels EM, Bijma HH, Galbally M, Bergink V. Lithium during pregnancy and after delivery: a review. Int J Bipolar Disord. 2018;6:26.

Preston JD, O'Neal JH, Talaga MC. Handbook of clinical psychopharmacology for therapists. 7th ed. Oacland (CA): New Harbinger Publications, Inc; 2013. p. 197–203.

Procyshyn R, Bezchlibnyk-Butler K, Jeffries J. Mood stabilizers. In: Clinical handbook of psychotropic drugs. 22nd ed. Goettingen (Germany): Hogrefe Publishing; 2017. p. 241–73.

Raja M. Lithium and kidney, 60 years later. Curr Drug Saf. 2011;6(5):291–303. https://doi.org/10.2174/157488611798918737.

Rosen MS. Lithium in child and adolescent bipolar disorder. Am J Psychiatry. 2017;12(2):3–5. https://doi.org/10.1176/appi.ajp-rj.2017.120202.

Taylor DM, Barnes RE, Young AH. Bipolar disorder. In: 13th, editor. The Maudsley prescribing guidelines in psychiatry. Hoboken (NY): John Wiley & Sons Ltd; 2017. p. 205–13.

Won E, Kim YK. An Oldie but Goodie: lithium in the treatment of bipolar disorder through neuroprotective and neurotrophic mechanisms. Int J Mol Sci. 2017;18(12):2679. https://doi.org/10.3390/ijms18122679.

Valproate

2

2.1   Clinical Case: Paola, a Patient with Bipolar Mania

Paola, a 63-year-old white female, presents to the emergency room, escorted by the police who found her wandering the streets at night. She wears a dirty skirt, an unbuttoned golf shirt, and appears older than her stated age. During the interview, she is restless and moderately agitated, and she makes puns and plays on words. Her sister, who came to the emergency room once she was called, reports that Paola has had a couple of weeks in which she has been "high," easily distracted, noisy, assertive, full of thoughts and ideas. She has not slept for days, stating that sleep is just a waste of time.

2.2   Family History

Paola's mother is 86-year-old, alive, and relatively healthy. Her father died at age 64 because of liver cancer. Her uncle spent long periods in a psychiatric hospital with a diagnosis of schizophrenia but with symptoms more consistent with a diagnosis of bipolar disorder with psychotic symptoms. Her sister is healthy. The patient graduated from college and works as an insurance agent.

© The Author(s), under exclusive license to Springer Nature Switzerland AG 2022
A. Fagiolini et al., *Pocket Guide to Practical Psychopharmacology*, https://doi.org/10.1007/978-3-030-98060-3_2

2.3   Clinical History

Paola has a history of bipolar disorder but recently stopped her lithium because of excessive tremor and because her primary care physician told her that it could be harmful to her psoriasis. Since she stopped lithium, she has had severe problems at work including a serious fight with her boss, which put her at high risk of being fired. She has some insight and is willing to take a new treatment but categorically refuses to re-start lithium.

2.4   Physical and Mental State Examination

Weight: 76 kg
   Height: 168 cm
   She is in menopause, appears older than stated age, and her grooming and hygiene are poor. Physical examination is otherwise unremarkable apart from psoriasis. She is disheveled and unkempt on presentation. She is agitated but establishes an acceptable rapport and is somewhat cooperative not difficult to redirect for interviewing, despite her inappropriate laughing and smiling. She is hyperverbal, speaks loudly, and fast, with a happy tone. Her self-esteem is increased but not to the point of being delusional. Attention and concentration are poor.

2.5   We Decide to Consider Starting Treatment with Valproate

2.5.1   What are the Indications of Valproate?

In most countries, valproate is indicated for the:

- Treatment of manic episodes associated with bipolar disorder
- Monotherapy and adjunctive therapy of complex partial seizures and simple and complex absence seizures
- Adjunctive therapy in patients with multiple seizure types that include absence seizures

- Prophylaxis of migraine headaches

  In the extended-release formulation, valproate is indicated for:

- Acute treatment of manic or mixed episodes associated with bipolar disorder, with or without psychotic features
- Monotherapy and adjunctive therapy of complex partial seizures and simple and complex absence seizures; adjunctive therapy in patients with multiple seizure types that include absence seizures
- Prophylaxis of migraine headaches

2.5.2   What are the Contraindications of Valproate?

- Patients with hepatic dysfunction shouldn't be prescribed with valproate

- Hypersensitivity to valproate or other ingredients used in the formulation

- For patients with urea cycle disorder, valproate is contraindicated

- Patients known to have mitochondrial (POLG; e.g., Alpers-Huttenlocher Syndrome) and children under two years of age who are suspected of having a POLG-related disorder

If risk-benefit evaluation favors use of valproate in pregnant patients, prophylactic administration of folic acid should be introduced.

2.5.3   What are the Warnings of Valproate?

- Liver toxicity, including fatalities, usually during the first 6 months of treatment. Children under the age of two years and patients with mitochondrial disorders are at higher risk. Monitor patients closely, and check serum liver testing prior to therapy and at frequent intervals thereafter.
- Teratogenicity, fetal risk, particularly neural tube defects, other major malformations, and decreased IQ.
- Pancreatitis, including fatal hemorrhagic cases.

2.6 What are the Precautions that You Should Keep in Mind When Prescribing Valproate?

- Cases of life-threatening pancreatitis have been reported in both children and adults receiving valproate.
- Valproate is associated with dose-related thrombocytopenia.
- Hyperammonemia has been reported in association with valproate therapy and may be present despite normal liver function tests. Patients with hyperammonemia may present symptoms that include lethargy, vomiting, changes in mental status, or hypothermia. May be more frequent when valproate is associated with topiramate.
- Drug Reaction with Eosinophilia and Systemic Symptoms (DRESS) has been reported in patients taking valproate.
- Antiepileptic drugs (AEDs), including valproate, may increase the risk of suicidal thoughts or behaviors.
- Valproate may stimulate the replication of the HIV and CMV viruses under certain experimental conditions.
- Children under the age of two years are at a considerably increased risk of developing fatal hepatotoxicity.
- Because of the risk to the fetus of decreased IQ, neurodevelopmental disorders, and major congenital malformations (including neural tube defects), valproate should not be used in pregnant women.

2.7 What is the Mechanism of Action of Valproate?

The exact mechanism of action is unknown. However, it has been suggested that valproate increases the brain concentrations of gamma-aminobutyric acid (GABA). Also, valproate has been associated with:

- •1   ☐Activation of extracellular signal-regulated kinase (ERK)

- •2   ☐Inhibition of γ-aminobutyric acid (GABA) catabolism

- •3   ☐Enhancement of brain-derived neurotrophic factor (BDNF)

- •4   ☐Decrease of protein kinase C

- •5   ☐Inhibition of inositol and thus blockage of voltage-gated sodium channels

- •6   ☐Anti-tumor activity by inhibition of histone deacetylase 1 (HDAC1) and other HDACs that potentially increases the expression of genes involved in apoptosis.

2.8   Which Laboratory Tests Would You Order for Paola?

Due to its hepatotoxic effects, valproate can increase liver enzymes. In some patients at the beginning or during chronic treatment with valproate, pancreatitis may occur. Therefore, to rule out hepatitis and pancreatitis, liver function tests and blood amylase levels have to be determined: Valproate may induce thrombocytopenia and, when thrombocytopenia is present, the medication should be discontinued.

At any sign of hyperammonemia (vomiting, lethargy, altered mental status), the treatment should be reconsidered.

Recommended baseline laboratory tests usually include:

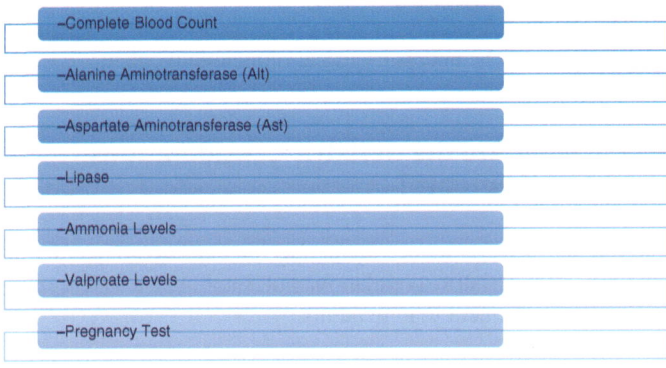

- –Complete Blood Count

- –Alanine Aminotransferase (Alt)

- –Aspartate Aminotransferase (Ast)

- –Lipase

- –Ammonia Levels

- –Valproate Levels

- –Pregnancy Test

2.9   Which Dose Would You Prescribe?

The recommended valproate initial dose for the treatment of mania is 750 mg daily. The dose should be increased as rapidly as possible to achieve the lowest therapeutic dose which produces the desired clinical effect or the desired range of plasma concentrations. The initial dose of valproate extended release is 25 mg/kg/day, increasing as rapidly as possible to achieve therapeutic response or desired plasma level, up to the maximum recommended dosage of 60 mg/kg/day.

2.10   Would You Consider Adjunctive Medications?

In clinical trials, valproate has been safely associated with lorazepam for patients with agitation, anxiety, or insomnia. For patients with psychotic symptoms or very severe agitation, a combination with an antipsychotic may be considered.

2.11   How Would You Monitor Paola's Tolerability and When Would You Repeat the Laboratory Tests?

Patients should be closely monitored for valproate tolerability. The baseline laboratory tests should be repeated after 3 days and then weekly or biweekly for one month, biweekly for another month, and then monthly or every 2–3 months. More frequent assessments may be necessary as per clinical judgement.

2.12   What Are the Geriatric Considerations for Valproate?

There is no strong evidence about specific considerations of valproate use in geriatric population, but somnolence and tremor may be more frequent than in adults.

Hypoalbuminemia in elderly patients can cause higher levels of free valproate and increased risk of parkinsonism (in those with dementia) and thrombocytopenia.

2.13   Can Valproate Be Used in Children and Adolescents?

- Children under the age of 2 are at higher risk of experiencing severe, life-threatening hepatic failure with valproate. The risk increases among children suffering from severe epilepsy or congenital metabolic disorder.
- Potentially fatal pancreatitis may occur in children treated with valproate. In case of gastrointestinal symptoms, pediatric patient has to be evaluated and drug administration has to be seized.
- In adolescents, valproate is frequently used in treatment of bipolar disorder, aggressive behavior as well as in migraine prophylaxis.
- In female adolescents, valproate use may lead to hyperandrogenism, delayed puberty, metabolic disorders, and decreased bone mineral density.

2.14   Can Valproate Be Used in Pregnant or Breastfeeding Women?

- Valproate is associated with congenital malformations such as neural tube defects and other structural abnormalities (e.g., craniofacial defects, cardiovascular malformations, hypospadias, limb malformations). The rate of malformations among children born to mothers using valproate is about four times higher than the rate among children born to epileptic mothers in treatment with other anti-seizure monotherapies. Folic acid supplementation prior to conception and during the first trimester of pregnancy decreases the risk for congenital neural tube defects in the general population. However, it is not known whether the risk of neural tube defects or decreased IQ in the children of women receiving valproate is reduced by folic acid supplementation. Nonetheless, dietary folic acid supplementation both prior to conception and during pregnancy should be routinely recommended for women using valproate.

- Because of the risk to the fetus of major malformations (including neural tube defects), decreased IQ, and neurodevelopmental disorders, valproate should not be administered to a woman of childbearing potential unless other medications have failed to provide adequate symptom control or are otherwise unacceptable.
- Breastfeeding while undergoing valproate treatment has not been proved to cause adverse effects in neonatal development. Between 1–10% of maternal plasma concentration can be found in breast milk.

2.15 What Would the Dose Be if Paola Had a Renal Disease?

A slight reduction (27%) in the clearance of valproate has been described in patients with renal failure (creatinine clearance < 10 mL/minute). However, no dosage adjustment appears to be necessary in these patients with renal failure. Protein binding in these patients is substantially reduced and therefore the monitoring total concentrations may be misleading.

2.16 What is the Pharmacokinetic Profile of Valproate?

The absorption of oral formulations of valproate takes place in gastrointestinal tract. The plasma protein binding of valproate is concentration dependent, and the free fraction increases from approximately 10% at 40 mcg/mL to 18.5% at 130 mcg/mL. Higher levels of free fraction can be found in elderly patients, those taking competitive protein-binding drugs, or those with hypoalbuminemia. In these cases, toxicity might develop despite normal serum levels.

The half-life ranges between 10–16 hours. Peak plasma concentrations are achieved 3–4 hours after orally administered valproate. At steady-state concentrations, valproate has linear pharmacokinetics within a dosage range of minimum 45–50 µg/mL.

2.17   What are the Most Common Interactions with Valproate?

- Medications that elevate levels of glucuronosyltransferases, may increase the clearance of valproate. For example, carbamazepine, and phenobarbital and ritonavir can double the clearance of valproate.

- Valproate has been found to be an inhibitor of some P450 isozymes, epoxide hydrase, and glucuronosyltransferases. For instance, a steady-state study, a 165% increase in the elimination half-life of lamotrigine was observed. The dose of lamotrigine should be reduced when co-administered with valproate.

- Since valproate inhibits glucuronidation, it may elevate plasma levels of certain drugs, including tricyclic antidepressants, anticonvulsants (lamotrigine), antipsychotics (quetiapine), anticoagulant warfarin and barbiturate phenobarbital.

- Carbapenem antibiotics (for example, ertapenem, imipenem, meropenem; this is not a complete list) may reduce serum valproate concentrations to subtherapeutic levels, resulting in loss of seizure control.

- Microsomal mediated oxidation is a relatively minor secondary metabolic pathway compared to glucuronidation and beta-oxidation. Hence, medications that inhibit P450 isozymes, usually have little effect on valproate clearance because cytochrome P450

- Concomitant administration of valproate and topiramate has been associated with hyperammonemia with and without encephalopathy

- Co-administration of valproate can affect the pharmacokinetics of other drugs (e.g. diazepam, ethosuximide, lamotrigine, phenytoin) by protein binding displacement or by inhibiting their metabolism

2.18   What are the Adverse Effects that You Would Monitor in a Patient like Paola?

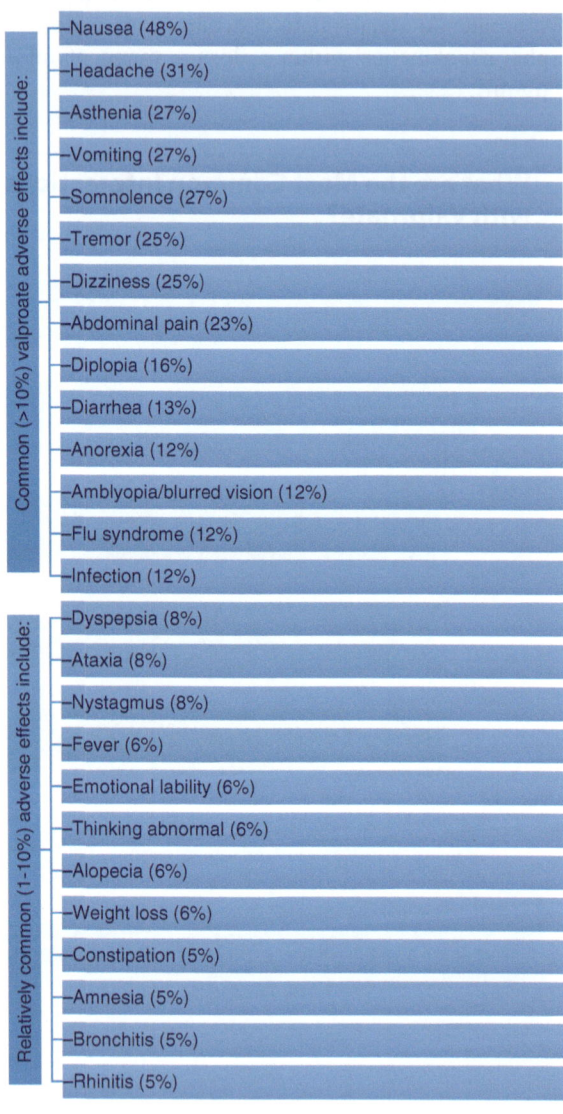

Common (>10%) valproate adverse effects include:

- Nausea (48%)
- Headache (31%)
- Asthenia (27%)
- Vomiting (27%)
- Somnolence (27%)
- Tremor (25%)
- Dizziness (25%)
- Abdominal pain (23%)
- Diplopia (16%)
- Diarrhea (13%)
- Anorexia (12%)
- Amblyopia/blurred vision (12%)
- Flu syndrome (12%)
- Infection (12%)

Relatively common (1-10%) adverse effects include:

- Dyspepsia (8%)
- Ataxia (8%)
- Nystagmus (8%)
- Fever (6%)
- Emotional lability (6%)
- Thinking abnormal (6%)
- Alopecia (6%)
- Weight loss (6%)
- Constipation (5%)
- Amnesia (5%)
- Bronchitis (5%)
- Rhinitis (5%)

2.19   Is There a Risk of Toxicity?

Acute intoxication may occur when plasma levels exceed normal values (50–125 mg/L).

- Excessive valproate doses (blood levels up to 150-1,500 mg/L) can cause heart rhythm abnormalities, respiratory depression, hematological, electrolyte or metabolic abnormalities. Signs of neurotoxicity can also be present. Seizure, cerebral edema, or coma can be fatal.
- Supportive therapy with L-carnitine is recommended.
- Antidotes for valproate toxicity are unavailable.

2.20   What Happens if Paola Abruptly Discontinues Valproate?

There is no strong evidence of worsening of bipolar symptoms after rapid discontinuation of valproate. However, the protection for recurring episodes is likely lost.

- There is no evidence of psychological or psychological dependence on anticonvulsants reported.
- Abrupt discontinuation of the drug, especially in patients with a seizure disorder, might provoke rebound seizures.

Further Reading

Ayano G. Bipolar disorders and valproate: pharmacokinetics, pharmacodynamics and therapeutic effects and indications of valproate: review of articles. Bipolar Disord. 2016;2:109. https://doi.org/10.4172/2472-1077.1000109.

Bowden CL. Valproate. In: Schatzberg A, Nemeroff C, editors. The American Psychiatric Association Publishing Textbook of Psychopharmacology. 5th ed. Washington (DC): The American Psychiatric Association Publishing; 2017. https://doi.org/10.1176/appi.books.9781615371624.

Depakene Prescribing information. https://www.accessdata.fda.gov/drugsatfda_docs/label/2009/018081s047,018082s032lbl.pdf

Depakote, FDA prescribing information. Last accessed on Sept 5 https://www.rxabbvie.com/pdf/depakote.pdf

Depakote ER, FDA prescribing information. Last accessed on Sept 5 https://www.rxabbvie.com/pdf/dep3.pdf

Maxmen JS, Kennedy SH, McIntyre RS. Psychotropic drugs fast facts. 4th ed. New York, New York: WW Norton & Co.; 2008. p. 260. ISBN: 978-0393-20529

Pope HG Jr, McElroy SL, Keck PE Jr, Hudson JI. Valproate in the treatment of acute mania. A placebo-controlled study. Arch Gen Psychiatry. 1991;48(1):62–8.

U. S. National Library of Medicine. Sodium valproate. https://pubchem.ncbi.nlm.nih.gov/compound/Depacon#section=Information-Sources

Valproic Acid Pathway, Pharmacodynamics. https://www.pharmgkb.org/pathway/PA165959313

Carbamazepine

3

3.1 Clinical Case: Claudio, a Young Patient with Bipolar Mania

Claudio is a 22-year-old male who presents to the outpatient unit accompanied by his father, who reports that the patient is experiencing severe distractibility, reduced sleep, irritability, racing thoughts, fluctuations from elevated to irritable mood, inflated self-esteem, and severe problems at school. That very morning, he was asked to leave a classroom after he started singing and dancing during a lecture.

3.2 Family History

Parents alive and divorced. The father is healthy and no history of mental disorder. The mother has a history of bipolar I disorder, alcoholism, and cocaine abuse. His sister is currently in treatment for borderline personality disorder. He has one elder brother in good physical and mental health. Claudio studies literature at the local university but has not taken any test in the previous 8 months because of his mood swings.

© The Author(s), under exclusive license to Springer Nature
Switzerland AG 2022
A. Fagiolini et al., *Pocket Guide to Practical Psychopharmacology*,
https://doi.org/10.1007/978-3-030-98060-3_3

3.3 Clinical History

Claudio has been treated for bipolar disorder since he was 13. He stopped lithium at age 20 because of treatment resistant polyuria. He was switched to valproate, which he stopped on his own because of nausea, tremor, and hair loss. He tried aripiprazole, quetiapine, and olanzapine, which he discontinued because of akathisia (aripiprazole), weight gain (olanzapine), sedation and hypotension (quetiapine).

3.4 Physical and Mental State Examination

Claudio is physically healthy but overweight. He is oriented and relatively cooperative. During the evaluation, mood quickly fluctuates from euphoric to irritable and vice versa. Shows brief and mild fluctuations towards depressive mood. Self-esteem is increased, with quasi-delusional traits of grandiosity. He acknowledges that he has not been his normal self for over a month. During the evaluation, he talks fast, laughs inappropriately, and spends most of the time describing his need to have sex several times a day and with as many people as possible. He is aware of the need to take medications but strongly refuses to consider the possibility of reinitiating lithium or valproate or any other medication that can give him sedation or akathisia.

3.5 We Decide to Consider Starting Treatment with Carbamazepine

3.5.1 What Are the Indications of Carbamazepine?

In many countries, carbamazepine is primarily indicated for partial seizures with complex symptomatology (psychomotor, temporal lobe), generalized tonic-clonic seizures (grand mal), mixed seizure patterns which include the above, or other partial or generalized seizures, pain associated with true trigeminal neuralgia.

In a number of countries, carbamazepine is also indicated for the treatment of acute manic or mixed episodes associated with bipolar I disorder.

3.5.2   What are the Contraindications of Carbamazepine?

Carbamazepine is contraindicated in patients with:

- Hypersensitivity to carbamazepine or other structurally related agent containing tricyclic component (e.g., amitriptyline) or any other formulation component
- Hepatic or cardiac rhythm disorders
- Bone-marrow depression
- Treatment with non-nucleoside reverse transcriptase inhibitors (because of the interaction with the cytochrome CYP3A4)

3.5.3   What are the Warnings of Carbamazepine?

- Serious dermatologic reactions

  Serious and possibly fatal dermatologic reactions including Stevens–Johnson syndrome (SJS) and toxic epidermal necrolysis (TEN) have been reported during treatment with carbamazepine. These adverse events are estimated to occur in 1–6 per 10,000 new users in countries with mainly Caucasian populations. However, the risk in certain Asian countries (i.e., Han Chinese) is estimated to be about 10 times higher. A strong association between the risk of developing SJS/TEN and the presence of HLA-b*1502, an inherited allelic variant of the hla-b gene, has been found in studies involving patients of Chinese ancestry or other ancestry, across broad areas of Asia. Patients with ancestry in genetically at-risk populations should be screened for the presence of HLA-b*1502 prior to initiating treatment with carbamazepine. Patients testing positive for the allele should not be treated with tegretol unless the benefit clearly outweighs the risk.

- Aplastic anemia and agranulocytosis
    Agranulocytosis and aplastic anemia have been reported in association with the use of carbamazepine. The risk of developing these reactions is 5–8 times greater for patients treated with carbamazepine than in the general population. The risk is approximately six patients per one million population per year for agranulocytosis and two patients per one million population per year for aplastic anemia.
- Transient or persistent decreased platelet or white blood cell counts are possible even if the majority of the cases of leukopenia have not progressed to the more serious conditions of aplastic anemia or agranulocytosis.

3.6   What are the Precautions that You Should Keep in Mind when Prescribing Carbamazepine?

- Given that hematological reactions may occur, patients should report any occurrence of bruising, petechial or purpuric hemorrhage, or ulceration. In such case, if leukocytes fall below 3000/mm^3, erythrocytes below 4×106/mm^3, and platelets below 100,000/mm^3, therapy has to be seized immediately.
- Carbamazepine interferes and enhances metabolism of drugs metabolized by CYP450. Therefore, if a female patient already using oral contraceptives is introduced with carbamazepine, alternative contraceptive methods should be considered.
- Asian patients with positive HLA-B*1502 should avoid carbamazepine administration, due to the risk of Stevens–Johnson syndrome or toxic epidermal necrolysis.
- Behavior changes, particularly suicidal thoughts, should be reported.
- There is evidence of tolerance to carbamazepine.
- If a soluble formulation is given at the same time with another liquid drug, insoluble precipitate may be formed.

3.7   Clinical Considerations

Our decision to prescribe carbamazepine was primarily based on his difficulty to tolerate other classic mood stabilizers and anti-psychotics.

3.8   What is the Mechanism of Action of Carbamazepine?

The exact mechanism of action of carbamazepine is unknown. Based on animal studies, the possible mechanisms of action include:

- Blockage of inactivated neuronal sodium channels, which leads to increased potassium and conductance
- Agonism with γ-aminobutyric acid (GABA) and thus enhancement of intracellular chloride accumulation
- Decrease of glutamate
- Increase of extracellular levels of serotonin

3.9   Which Laboratory Tests Would You Order for Claudio?

Before starting carbamazepine, it is recommended to check:

- Complete Blood Count (CBC)
- Serum electrolytes (watch for hyponatremia)
- Blood urea nitrogen
- Creatinine
- Hepatic enzymes
- HLA-b*1502 typing for patients at risk
- Pancreatic enzymes
- Pregnancy test
  - When risk of osteopenia exists, bone density should be determined.

3.10   Which Dose Would You Prescribe?

> **Dosing for adults with acute mania are the following:**
>
> - Extended-release capsule 200 mg initially twice a day, then daily increase of 200 mg to achieve a maximum of 1,600 mg/day
> - With immediate-release formulations, daily dosage starts at 200 mg twice a day and then ranges from 800-1,600 mg, based on blood levels and tolerability, divided in 3-4 daily doses

> **•For adults with trigeminal neuralgia:**
>
> - 100 mg tablets twice a day or 50 mg oral suspensions 4 times a day and increase by up to 200 mg/day, to a maximum dose of 1,200 mg/day or maintenance dose of 400-800 mg/day.

> **For adults with epilepsy:**
>
> - Initially 200 mg twice a day tablets or 100 mg 4 times a day oral suspension. Then weekly increase of 200 mg per day up to maximum dose of 1,600 m/day or maintenance dose of 800-1,200 mg/day [19]

> **For children with epilepsy:**
>
> - Below 6 years–initially 10-20 mg/kg per day divided in 2-3 doses for immediate-release tables or in 4 doses for oral suspension or every 12 hours for extended-release formulations. Then weekly increase doses up to maximum of 35 kg/mg/day
> - 6-12 years of age: 100 mg twice a day tablets, or capsules, or 100 mg 4 times s a day oral suspension. Then weekly increase of 100 mg per day up to maximum dose of 1,000 m/day or maintenance dose of 400-800 mg/day
> - Over 12 years of age: 200 mg twice a day tablets, or capsules, or 100 mg 4 times s a day oral suspension. Then weekly increase of 200 mg per day up to maximum dose of 1,000 m/day (12-15 years) or 1,200 mg/day (older than 15 years) or maintenance dose of 800-1,200 mg/day.

3.11   How Would You Monitor Claudio's Tolerability and When Would You Repeat the Laboratory Tests?

- Follow-up laboratory analyses and carbamazepine blood concentrations may be repeated after 5–10 days, then every two weeks for 1–2 months, than monthly, every 2–3 months or more frequently if clinically indicated.

3.12   What if Claudio was an Older Patient?

- Gradual dosing should be established in the elderly and those with liver damage.
- Although appropriate studies on the relationship of age to the effects of carbamazepine have not been performed in the geri-

atric population, it is known that elderly patients are more likely to have confusion or agitation, which requires caution and may require to discontinue or adjust the dose of carbamazepine.

- Elderly patients with history of cardiovascular diseases should be monitored.
- Carbamazepine in elderly can frequently lead to hyponatremia.

3.13   Can Carbamazepine be Used in Children and Adolescents?

- Carbamazepine has been used in children with seizures disorders or behavior disorders.
- The medication has not been widely studied in children and adolescents, especially for the long-term adverse effects. Children are at higher risk of experiencing major toxicities.

3.14   Can Carbamazepine Be Used in Pregnant Patients?

Carbamazepine can produce teratogenic effects if administered during pregnancy; teratogenic effects are worsening in combined anticonvulsant therapy. When administered during pregnancy, developmental delay in infants may occur.

- Breastfeeding while undergoing carbamazepine treatment should be discontinued because harmful epoxide metabolite can be transferred to breast milk.

3.15   What Would the Dose Be if Claudio Had a Renal Disease:

- If glomerular filtration rate is <10 mL/min: Administer 75% of dose and monitor
- If the patient receives peritoneal dialysis and hemodialysis: Administer 75% of dose and monitor

3.16   How about if Claudio Had a Liver Disease?

- Use caution or consider using a different medication, as is metabolized primarily in the liver

3.17   What is the Pharmacokinetic Profile of Carbamazepine?

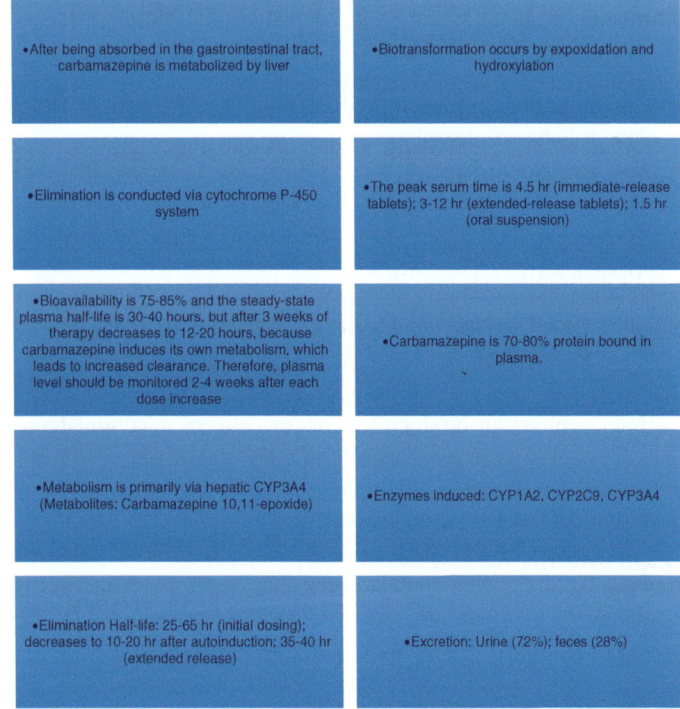

3.18 What are the Pharmacokinetic Interactions of Carbamazepine?

• Carbamazepine induces catabolic enzymes (including CYP3A4) and thus lowers the serum concentrations or various agents

• Carbamazepine can decrease plasma levels of certain antidepressants, anticonvulsants, dihydropyridine CCBs, antipsychotics, muscle relaxants, immunosuppressants, analgesics, anxiolytics, steroids, anticoagulants and anti-infective agents.

• Decrease in thyroxine and estrogens during carbamazepine treatment also might occur.

• Inhibitors of CYP3A4 increase plasma levels of carbamazepine and may lead to toxicity:

☐ Calcium channel blockers (verapamil, diltiazem)
☐ Antibiotics (erythromycin)
☐ Antifungal agents (fluconazole)
☐ Histamine H_2 receptor antagonist (cimetidine)

Some drugs within SSSRIs.

3.19 Pharmacogenomics

HLA-B*1502

- When taking carbamazepine, 1 in 20 patients with HLA-B*1502 will have a severe dermatologic reaction, e.g., toxic epidermal necrolysis (TEN) or Stevens–Johnson syndrome (SJS).
- This allele occurs almost exclusively in patients with ancestry across broad areas of Asia, including Malaysians, Han Chinese, South Asian Indians, Thais, and Filipinos.

HLA-A*3101

- Patients of European, Japanese, and Korean ancestry may develop hypersensitivity reactions when using carbamazepine and this may be linked to the presence of HLA-A*3101 gene. These reactions include SJS and TEN.
- HLA-A*3101 is carried by more than 15% of patients of Native American, Japanese, Southern Indian, and Arabic ancestry; up to about 10% in patients of European, Han Chinese, Latin American, Korean, and Indian ancestry; and up to about 5% in African-Americans and patients of Thai, Chinese (Hong Kong), and Taiwanese ancestry.

3.20   What are the Adverse Effects that You Would Monitor in a Patient like Claudio?

Carbamazepine use may cause several adverse effects, including:

- Neurotoxicity—sedation, lethargy, ataxia, diplopia, nystagmus, cognitive or behavioral changes.
- Hematological changes such as decreased number of white blood cells and platelets. Although rarely, malignant aplastic anemia can happen.
- Changes in electrolytes (hyponatremia).
- Hepatic changes—elevated values of transaminases.
- GI changes—nausea.
- Endocrine—weight gain.
- Dermatological—rash; rarely, toxic epidermal necrolysis and Stevens–Johnson syndrome may occur. The risk is estimated to be about 1–6 per 10,000 new users in countries with mainly Caucasian populations. However, the risk in some Asian countries is estimated to be about 10 times higher. Carbamazepine should be discontinued at the first sign of a rash, unless the rash is clearly unrelated to this medication. If signs or symptoms suggest SJS/TEN, use of this drug should not be resumed and alternative therapy should be considered.

- Menstrual cycle disturbances, including polycystic ovaries.
- Increased risk of suicidality.

Frequent (>10%) side effects include:

Ataxia (15%)
Dizziness (44%)
Drowsiness (32%)
Nausea (29%)
Vomiting (18%)

Relatively frequent (1–10%) side effects include dry mouth (8%).

3.21   What if Claudio Develops Toxicity?

•Carbamazepine toxic effects usually occurs if plasma levels exceed 50 mmol/L in adults	•Children are at greater risk of drug toxicity because of overproduction of toxic epoxide products	•Symptoms of carbamazepine overdose usually occur 1-3 hours after drug ingestion
•Patients may experience dizziness, irregular heart rhythm, drowsiness, generalized seizure, disorientation, stupor or coma	•Anticholinergic symptoms are also common	•Antidotes for carbamazepine toxicity are unavailable and the treatment is symptomatic

3.22   What Happens if Claudio Discontinues Carbamazepine?

- There are isolated cases reported of depression and mood disorder exacerbation, respectively, after treatment discontinuation.
- Abrupt discontinuation of the drug, especially in patients with a seizure disorder, might provoke rebound seizures.

Further Reading

Carbamazepine. Medscape. Last accessed at https://reference.medscape.com/drug/tegretol-xr-equetro-carbamazepine-343005 on Sept 10, 2022

Carbamazepine, Tegretol FDA prescribing information. Last accessed on Sept 4, 2021: https://www.accessdata.fda.gov/drugsatfda_docs/label/2009/016608s101,018281s048lbl.pdf

Carbamazepine Extended-Release Capsules, Equetro FDA prescribing information. Last accessed on Sept 4, 2021 https://www.accessdata.fda.gov/drugsatfda_docs/label/2009/021710s006lbl.pdf

Maxmen JS, Kennedy SH, McIntyre RS. In: Jerrold S, editor. Psychotropic drugs fast facts. 4th ed. New York, New York: WW Norton & Co.; 2008. p. 260. ISBN: 978-0393-20529.

Procyshyn R, Bezchlibnyk-Butler K, Jeffries J. Mood stabilizers. In: Clinical handbook of psychotropic drugs. 22nd ed. Goettingen (Germany): Hogrefe Publishing; 2017. p. 241.